Bad Breath Natural Cure

Powerful Methods to Boost Mouth Freshness, Achieve Excellent Breath, And Improve Confidence

By

Kim Hilton

Bad Breath Natural Cure

First edition. July, 2018.

Copyright © 2018 Kim Hilton

Written by Kim Hilton

Books by The Same Author

- <u>Boost Your Energy Levels: 60 Natural Ways to Get Rid of Fatigue, Dizziness, Weakness, And Lack of Motivation</u>

- <u>How to Get Rid Of Stretch Marks Naturally</u>

- <u>How to Break Sugar Cravings with Nutritional Supplements: Healthy and Natural Alternatives</u>

- <u>The Anti-Anxiety Cookbook: Nutritional Plan to Cure Depression and Anxiety (Stress Relief and Mental Health Cookpot)</u>

- <u>Eating Disorder Recovery Workbook: How to Recover from</u>

Table of Contents

Introduction

Bad breath or mouth odor medically referred to as fetor oris or halitosis is an embarrassing condition that can have a toll on one's health, self-esteem and, confidence. Medically, the first symptom of bad breath is the unpleasant mouth odor that is often recognized by a third-party instead of the individual.

It is estimated that 25% of the global population have mouth odor (one in every four persons has mouth odor) and it is mostly caused by poor dental hygiene. It is the third most common cause for visits to the dentist office, the first is tooth decay followed by gum disease.

It can be induced by the presence of bacteria in the mouth, poor dental hygiene and it can be a sign of an underlying health condition, indigestion and digestive problems. Excessive consumption of junk food and other evidences of an unhealthy lifestyle are also causes of bad breath.

"Since the foods eaten are broken in the mouth, it is only obvious to say that digestion starts in the mouth."

Strongly scented foods like garlic and onions leave their scent in your mouth even after brushing, washing your tongue, and flossing.

"The unpleasant smell only fades away when the foods eaten are able to move completely out of the body."

Poor dental hygiene allows the growth and multiplication of bacteria in the mouth because food particles will be left in your mouth, on your tongue and between your teeth. These microbes will feed on them and multiply, and, this, in turn, will cause bad breath.

PS: Bad breath rarely occurs in babies but when it does, it is a sign of an undiagnosed illness or infection and the baby should be treated immediately.

Causes of Bad Breath

- Breathing through the mouth:

"This is among the common causes of bad breath as breathing with your mouth often leads to dryness of the mouth, where it naturally supposed to be wet. It dries up saliva which is needed to neutralize acids produced by plaque and to moisten the mouth."

The consistent and continuous flow of saliva within the mouth are is essential as it functions in cleaning up dead cells from the gums, tongue and inner cheeks.

If there is no much saliva to do these,

bacteria and dead cells will accumulate

and decompose, resulting in a bad breath.

Additionally, dry mouth might be caused

by some prescribed medication or

impaired salivary glands. This is to say

that handful of medications prescribed

can directly cause dehydration which

also amounts to the dryness of the mouth.

Natural causes of dryness might include

mode of feeding, rate of hydration and

habitual breathing through the mouth.

- Oral infections

- Morning breath because the secretion of saliva is reduced while you sleep.

- Objects stuck in one's nose or obstructed nostrils

- Eating strongly scented foods or smelly foods

- Dentures and braces

- Fasting and skipping meals leads to less production of saliva

- Large doses of vitamin supplements

- Smoking; this unhealthy habit leads to dry mouth and it also increases the number of compounds that cause odor in your mouth, lungs and respiratory system.

- Some medications like antihistamines, paraldehyde, triamterene, and diuretics cause mouth odor as side effects, they cause dry mouth.

- Alcoholism

- Buildup of plaques and cavities

- A low-carb diet causes halitosis

- Pregnancy: vomiting and nausea, dehydration, eating lots of foods and hormonal changes can cause mouth odor in pregnant women.

Signs and Symptoms of Bad Breath

- An unpleasant odor from your mouth is the most obvious and accurate sign of bad breath

- A white or colored coating on your tongue

- An unpleasant taste or sour taste or changes in the way you taste things

- Dry mouth

Health Conditions Associated with Bad Breath

"Persistent or chronic bad breath may be a warning or telltale sign of a health condition."

Some of the conditions associated with bad breath are:

• Gum disease (caused by the accumulation of plaque on the teeth), untreated gum disease can damage the jawbones and gums and it raises the risks of heart disease.

•   Oral thrush or yeast infection of the mouth

•   Ketoacidosis

•   Cavities (dental caries)

•   Allergies

•   Xerostomia, also known as dry mouth

•   Sjogren's syndrome, an autoimmune disease that occurs in young women, women with this condition have a very dry mouth which leads to halitosis.

•   Diabetes

- Kidney problems

- Chronic sinus infections

- Stomach and peptic ulcers

- Liver problems

- Obstruction of the bowels

- Bronchitis, pneumonia and other respiratory tract infections

- Postnasal drips

- Chronic acid reflux

- Digestive problems

- Sore throats

- •	Throat infections

- •	Lactose intolerance

How to Prevent Bad Breath

• Practice good and proper oral hygiene

• Brush twice daily, in the morning and at night when you want to go to bed

• Brush or scrub your tongue when you brush your teeth

• Change your toothbrush after two or three months

• Remove dentures at night before you sleep and clean them thoroughly in the morning before putting them back.

- Go for dental checkup once a year

- Quit smoking or using tobacco products like tobacco chewing gum.

- Drink lots of water daily to keep the mouth hydrated and clean

Natural Remedies for Bad Breath

The main cure or remedy for halitosis is to find the root cause and address it, whether it is caused by a medical condition or bad oral hygiene. When the root cause is corrected, the condition can be easily reversed.

Below are effective home treatments you can use while treating the root cause of bad breath or correcting unhealthy lifestyles.

Proper Hydration

Quality hydration is an effective yet simple remedy for bad breath, it flushes away bad microbes and food particles and keeps the mouth clean and moist and it keeps your breath odorless and fresh.

After eating, swish water in your mouth for a while, this will remove food particles and keep it clean. Also, you should drink lots of water during the day.

Eucalyptus Oil

This essential oil has a strong antibacterial and bactericidal effect on a wide range of bacteria. It treats pains and swellings in the mouth due to its analgesic and anti-inflammatory effects.

Add three or four drops of eucalyptus essential oil into a glass of water and gargle with this. Rinse your mouth with water when you are done. Do this once daily until you see an improvement.

Baking Soda

This powerful remedy fight mouth odor by killing bacteria in the mouth, it also corrects the pH and levels of acids in the mouth thereby getting rid of bad breath.

Add a teaspoon of baking soda to a cup of clean water and use this solution as a mouth rinse. It kills oral bacteria and eliminates them. Do this daily.

Try and brush your teeth with baking soda two times every week to reduce high levels of acids present in the mouth and to also fight the formation of plaque. All these can cause bad breath, it also stops bacteria from accumulating on your tongue.

Ginger

Ginger is a great therapy for bad breath because it has powerful antimicrobial, antibacterial properties, it kills harmful bacteria that cause mouth odor and other oral problems.

It also treats throat and mouth infections and it keeps oral cancers at bay when taken regularly. You can chew on fresh ginger root and you can take ginger tea many times daily.

Although ginger should be avoided especially among individual with prescribed medications for blood thinning, it can be used as a mouth rinse or to be added excessively in teas.

Apple Cider Vinegar

Raw, unfiltered and organic apple cider vinegar fights bad breath by killing the bacteria responsible for this and by fighting acidity too because it alkalizes the body.

Add one tablespoon of ACV inside a cup of water and gargle with it, do this three times every day. You can also drink this solution before each meal, this will boost healthy digestion and prevent bad breath caused by indigestion and other digestive problems.

Grapefruit Seed Extract

This citrus fruit fights mouth odor, it also kills bacteria because it has antimicrobial properties. It stops their growth and activities and deodorizes your mouth.

Add two drops of grapefruit seed extract to your toothbrush and gently brush your teeth with it. Rinse your mouth with clean water afterward and do this once daily.

This remedy is so effective that you will see an improvement in one week.

Fennel

Fennel seeds are natural mouth fresheners with an excellent result. It has powerful antiseptic and antibacterial properties that kill bacteria in the mouth and it effectively control bad breath.

Consume fennel tea many times daily, steep 2 teaspoons of fennel seeds inside a cup of hot water for ten minutes; that is how you make fennel tea. You may also chew fresh fennel seeds, this will boost your production of saliva and freshen your breath also.

Salt Water

This is a simple but effective home remedy for bad breath, it kills harmful microbes in the mouth. It neutralizes high acidity in the mouth and keeps the mouth clean and free of bacteria.

"Mix a glass of water with a tablespoonful of table salt.

Stir in order to mix well.

Gargle the mixture until finished."

The procedure should be repeated twice a day.

Tea Tree Oil

This is a strong natural disinfectant, its strong antiseptic properties kills a host of microbes including bacteria that cause bad breath.

Add tea tree essential oil to your toothpaste and use it to brush your teeth and scrub your tongue on a daily basis. You can make an effective mouth wash that can expel bad breath using tea tree oil.

"Add the following mixture in a glass of water:

- Peppermint oil (3 drops)

- Lemon oil (3 drops)

- Tea tree essential oil (3 drops)"

"Use this solution to wash your mouth three times daily."

Studies have proved the workability of these mixture in getting rid of bad breath.

Sesame Oil

This cleanses the mouth and improves your general dental health just like coconut oil. It has antimicrobial property and it also whitens the teeth.

Add a teaspoon of sesame oil to a cup of water and swish this solution around your mouth for a few minutes, make sure it touches all corners of your mouth.

Spit it out, don't swallow it and then gargle with lukewarm water. This should be done every morning and you will see improvement.

Cinnamon

There is an active compound in this herb called cinnamic aldehyde, it kills bacteria in the mouth because it is an antibacterial and antiseptic compound and it masks bad breath.

Boil some teaspoons of cinnamon powder in one cup of water, you can add cardamom and bay leaves. Let the solution get warm, and then you strain it and drink. Do this many times every day.

This herbal tea should also be used as a mouth wash to freshen your breath and expel bacteria from the mouth.

Unripe Guava

Unripe guava is a powerful remedy for a lot of oral problems like bleeding gums, mouth odor, diseased gums, sensitive teeth and tooth decay.

It contains lots of vital nutrients that boost healthy dental health. It contains tannic acids, ascorbic acid, oxalate and malic acid. Eat unripe guava to fight mouth odor and to boost your dental health.

Herbal Teas

Both green and black teas contain lots of antioxidants and antiseptic compounds that kill bacteria in the mouth and cure bad breath. Other herbal teas like sage, peppermint, mint, clove and others all help reverse this condition and kill the microbes causing bad breath.

Drink any of this herbal teas many times daily. This will help keep your breath fresh.

Cardamom

Indians have for centuries used this spice to fight bad breath, they take it after meals, it is a natural mouth freshener, and it deodorizes your mouth thereby fighting bad breath.

It masks halitosis with its fragrance. After eating foods with strong scents like onions or garlic, chew on few pods of cardamom, this will mask the odor and freshen your breath.

You can eat the whole pod or you eat only the seeds inside.

Fenugreek

Fenugreek tea is highly effective in treating bad breath induced by catarrhal infections. Take fenugreek tea many times daily until you notice an improvement.

Zinc

This vital mineral boosts oral health. Studies have linked deficiency in zinc to mouth odor, it kills harmful bacteria and keeps the mouth clean and free from microbes.

Natural sources of zinc are dark green leafy vegetables, pumpkin seeds, cacao, seeds and nuts and gourd; organ meats are also good sources of zinc.

In chronic and severe cases of mouth odor, your doctor can prescribe zinc supplements for you. Please, take it according to prescription to avoid toxicity.

Zinc also fortify the immune system and improves the general health of your body.

Activated Charcoal

Activated charcoal helps eliminate impurities and bacteria in your mouth. It kills harmful microbes, fights the formation of plaque and it even whitens the teeth.

Put ½ teaspoon of this activated charcoal on your toothbrush and use this in brushing your teeth. Ensure you also scrub your tongue, use large amount of water to rinse your mouth thoroughly to get rid of all the activated charcoal.

Do this three times every week until the bad breath is eliminated.

Probiotics

Probiotics prevent digestive problems which cause bad breath and they also kill harmful microbes in the body.

They fight indigestion, constipation, heart burn, sluggish digestive system, and other digestive disorders that cause heart burn and they effectively treat bad breath caused by poor nutrition and excessive and indecriminate use of antibiotics.

Indigestion and other digestive problems create lots of gas in your body and some of these gases are expelled through your mouth and, this, in turn, will lead to bad breath.

Probiotics fight and replace harmful microbe in the mouth that cause mouth odor and they also eliminate volatile sulfur compounds that cause bad breath.

Rich sources of probiotics are fermented foods like yogurt, kefir, kombucha tea, sauerkraut and other fermented grains, fruits and vegetables.

Probiotics are also available in capsules and supplements. Take probiotics daily to reverse bad breath.

Cloves

The antibacterial and antiseptic properties of this herb makes them effective in treating mouth odor, they kill harmful microbes and freshen your breath. Chew few pieces of cloves daily to get rid of bad breath in a short time.

Clove tea is also effective and very easy to make. Boil a good quantity of cloves in one cup of water and let it get warm.

Strain the solution and drink, you can also make use of it as a mouthwash. Do this two times every day.

Peppermint

Peppermint tea and peppermint essential oil are powerful remedies for bad breath. It has antimicrobial and antiseptic properties.

 "The bacteria mostly responsible for causing bad breath in humans and animals can be easily eliminated using peppermint."

Additionally, it provides the pleasant freshness to improve your confidence being assured that you have a clean mouth.

It has a nice scent that helps in masking bad breath and studies have shown that it is more effective than chemical mouth rinse. Add three or more drops of this essential oil inside a cup of water use it to gargle.

You can also drink peppermint tea many times daily and this herbal tea can also be used a mouth rinse. Rinse your mouth with peppermint tea at least three times every day till you notice an improvement.

Sugar-free Gums

This is an effective remedy for halitosis, it increases the production and low of saliva in the mouth. Apart from the provision of clean and fresh breath, sugar-free gums help in keeping the mouth moisturized and well aerated, therefore getting rid of bad breath.

Use sugar-free gums because bacteria feed on sugar and excess sugar can cause tooth decay, cavities and a weak defense system. Use natural gums that contain mint, peppermint or other strong herbs that can help you eliminate bad breath

Sage

This ancient herb is a strong remedy for halitosis. Studies have proven its effectiveness against a wide range of microbes that cause bad breath like Porphyromonas gingivalis, Streptococcus mutans, and Candida albicans.

Take sage tea twice daily and you can use it as a mouth rinse. Rinse your mouth with sage tea three times daily. Continue until you see results.

Parsley

Parsley contains a rich amount of chlorophyll which is responsible for its green colour. This compound, chlorophyll neutralizes bad breath and keeps the mouth clean, fresh and microbe-free.

Chew on fresh parsley leaves if you can, you can dip it in apple cider vinegar and chew it to boost its effectiveness. You can make smoothies with parsley or juice it and sip the juice regularly to refresh your breath and fight bad breath.

It aids healthy digestion and prevent indigestion, heartburn, acid reflux and other digestive problems which cause bad breath.

Coconut Oil

Coconut oil kills bacteria and other harmful microbes, it keeps the mouth clean and free of microbes thereby fighting bad breath. Take two tablespoons of pure coconut oil two times daily till you notice an improvement.

You should also swish coconut oil in your mouth for ten minutes. Swish it very well and make sure it touches all nook and crannies of your mouth and then you spit it out. Rinse your mouth afterward. Do this three times daily.

Lemon Juice

This home remedy has been used or the past one thousand years as a standard herbal cure for bad breath, even among different other recipes. Their rich content of acids kill bacteria and other germs that cause mouth odor. It prevents the growth of bacteria and puts a stop to their activities.

It also has a sweet and strong scent that covers or masks the unpleasant odor in the mouth. Don't take lemon juice every day, it can destroy your enamel, it is safer to dilute it with equal amount of water, this forms lemon water, which can be used as a mouth wash and you can also drink it regularly.

Regular intake of lemon water stops bad breath and it also prevents digestive problems which is a major cause of halitosis. You can add a pinch of table salt your lemon water to boosts it bacteria killing property and to increase the production of saliva, thus fighting a dry mouth at the same time.

Epsom Salt

Epsom salt is a detoxifying substance used in its natural form to get rid of toxins form the body. with it antibacterial properties, it helps in providing a conducive environment for the positive bacteria. This helps it to keep the mouth clean and free of microbes and thereby treat mouth odor.

Add a teaspoon of Epsom salt to a cup of lukewarm water and gargle with it. Do every day and when you notice an improvement, skip a day by doing it alternatively.

When to See a Doctor

If proper hygiene and all these remedies don't eliminate bad breath and you notice the following symptoms, then you need to see a doctor so that he can rule out any serious infection or commence treatment immediately.

- A high body temperature

- Fatigue

- Persistent dry mouth

- White spots on your tonsils

- •	The presence of sores in your mouth

- •	Dental pain

- •	Broken tooth or tooth decay

- •	Experiencing pain and difficulty when swallowing or chewing

Books by The Same Author

- <u>Boost Your Energy Levels: 60 Natural Ways to Get Rid of Fatigue, Dizziness, Weakness, And Lack of Motivation</u>

- <u>How to Get Rid Of Stretch Marks Naturally</u>

- <u>How to Break Sugar Cravings with Nutritional Supplements: Healthy and Natural Alternatives</u>

- <u>The Anti-Anxiety Cookbook: Nutritional Plan to Cure Depression and Anxiety (Stress Relief and Mental Health Cookpot)</u>

- <u>Eating Disorder Recovery Workbook: How to Recover from Eating Disorder On Your Own (Anorexia, Bulimia Nervosa, And Binge Eating)</u>
- <u>100 Health Hacks Nobody Ever Told You: Natural Tips and Tricks for Enhanced and Prudent Well-Being</u>
- <u>How to Lower Blood Pressure Naturally & Quickly: Powerful Tricks to Deal with Hypertension Using Supplements and Other Natural Remedies</u>
- <u>Reverse Type 2 Diabetes: How to Control and Prevent Diabetes Naturally</u>

www.ingramcontent.com/pod-product-compliance
Lightning Source LLC
Chambersburg PA
CBHW031428250726

48656CB00002B/877